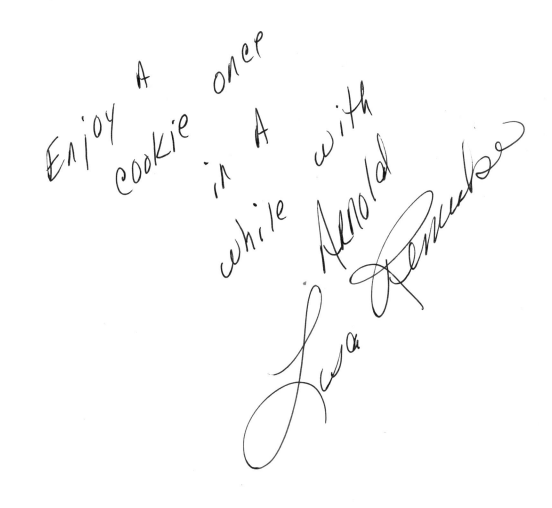

Enjoy A once
cookie in A
while with
Arnold

Lisa Remenbe

Written by Lisa (Mimi) Reinicke

Illustrated by Stephen Reinicke

Mimi's son, of whom she is terrifically proud.

Special thanks to Mike Hamel for his editing expertise

Thank you to Delon at Sunrise Printing and Design Company. You are amazing to work with

An extra thank you to Rich Reinicke
for juggling 5 things at once to make this happen.

For all children who love animals, especially cute little pigs.

ISBN 978-0-9978103-0-1

Printed in China

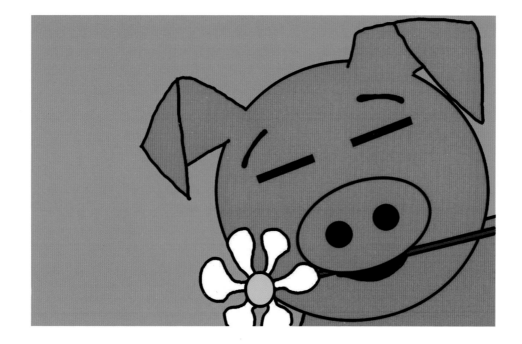

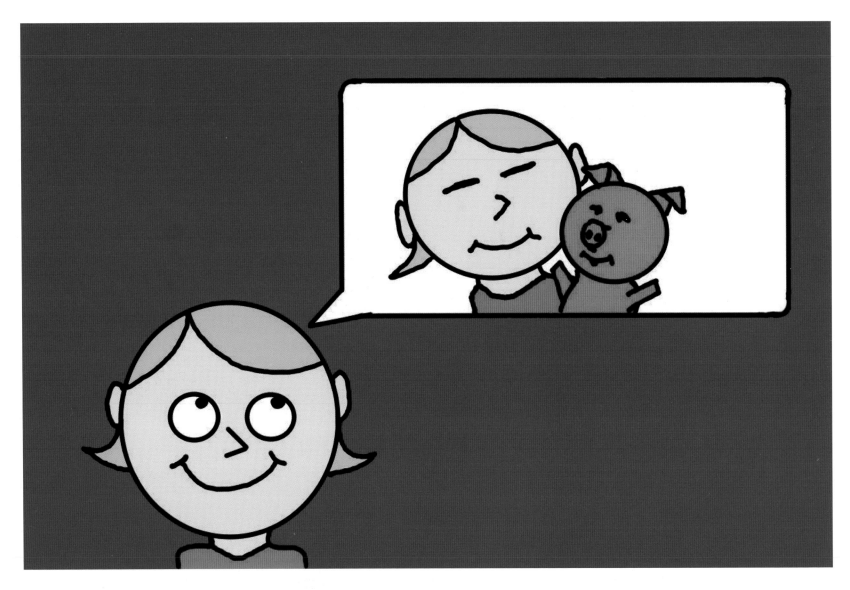

On Mother's Day our Mom wanted a pig for a present. Her two little boys found a cute little pig with personality to give her.

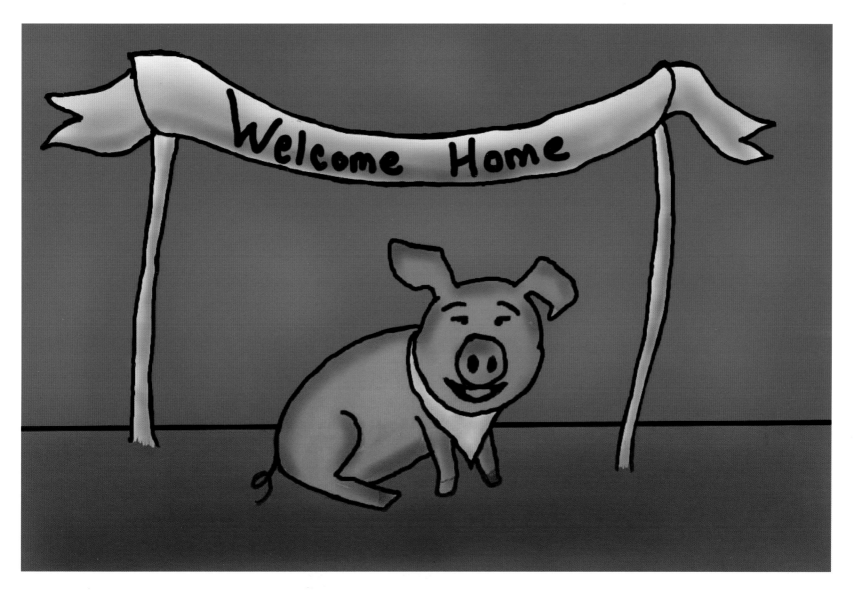

She welcomed the cute little pig into our home and named him Arnold. He was so tiny and round. He was sweet and pink and made the cutest little oink sound as he ran.

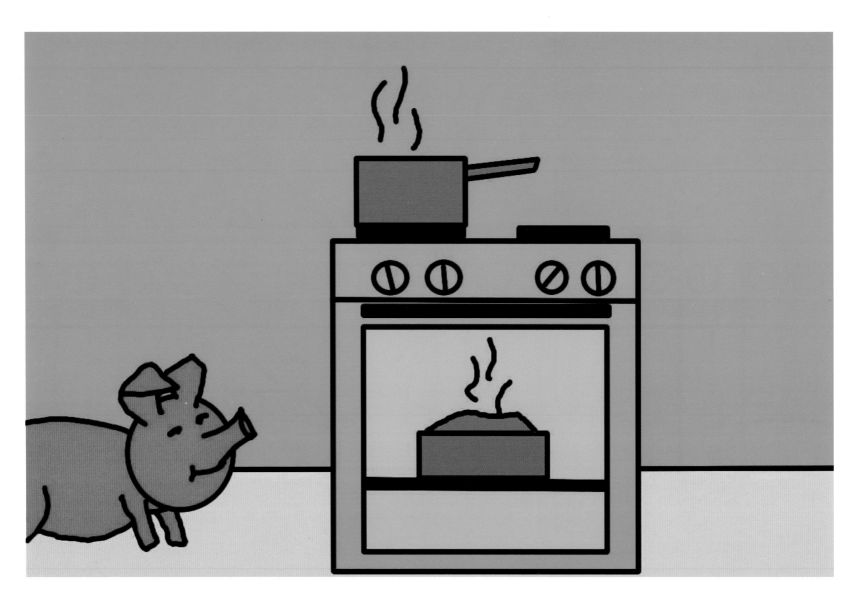

Mom soon learned that not only did Arnold have a great personality, but he also had a great appetite. He was hungry all the time!

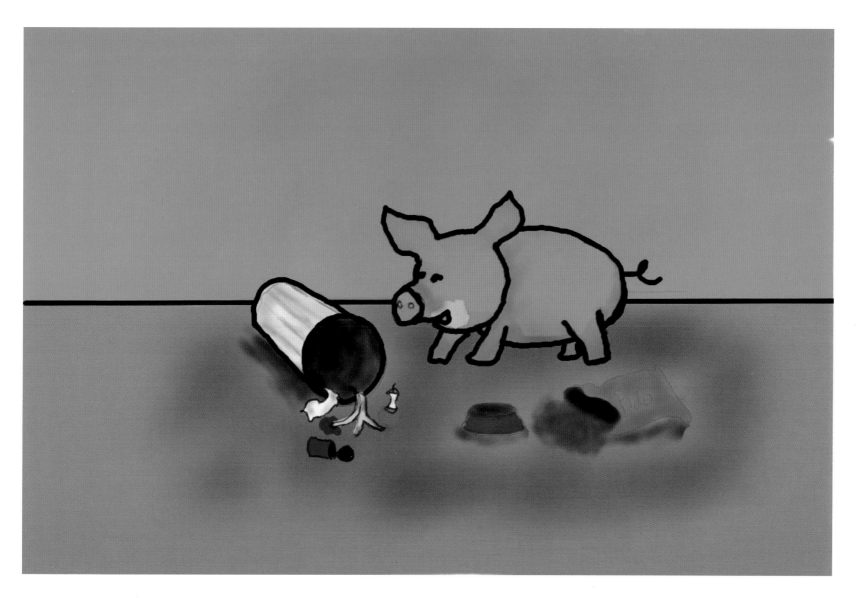

Arnold was always after food. He would eat all of the dog's food. He would eat all of the baby's food. Most of all, he loved to eat trash.

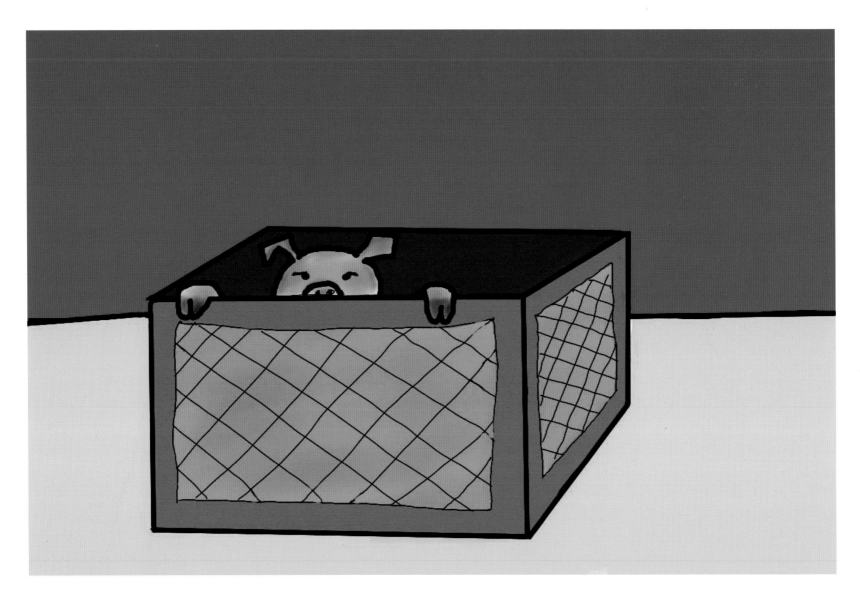

At first, Mom would keep Arnold in a play pen so he couldn't get into all the food that wasn't made for cute little piggies.

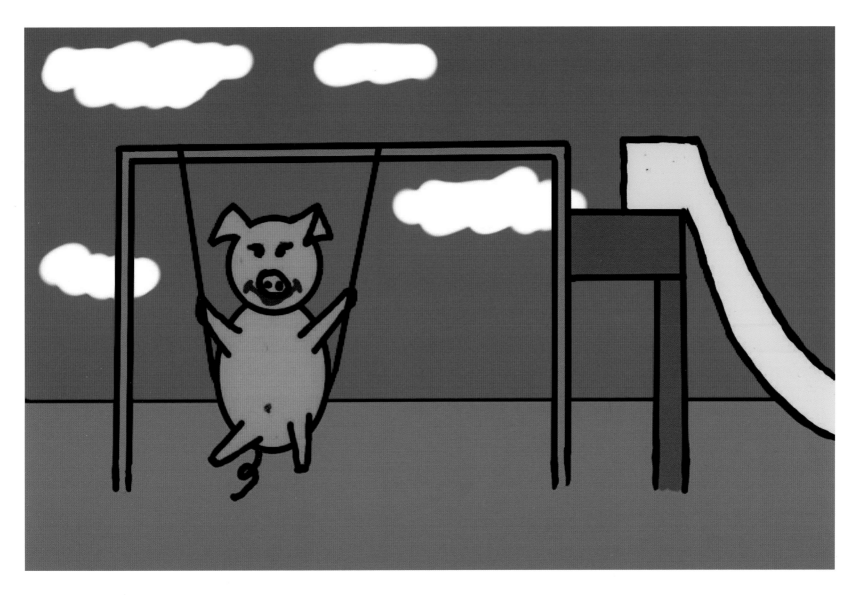

As Arnold grew, he would not fit in the play pen anymore, so he was sent to the yard to play where he would sing his oink song and play all day long.

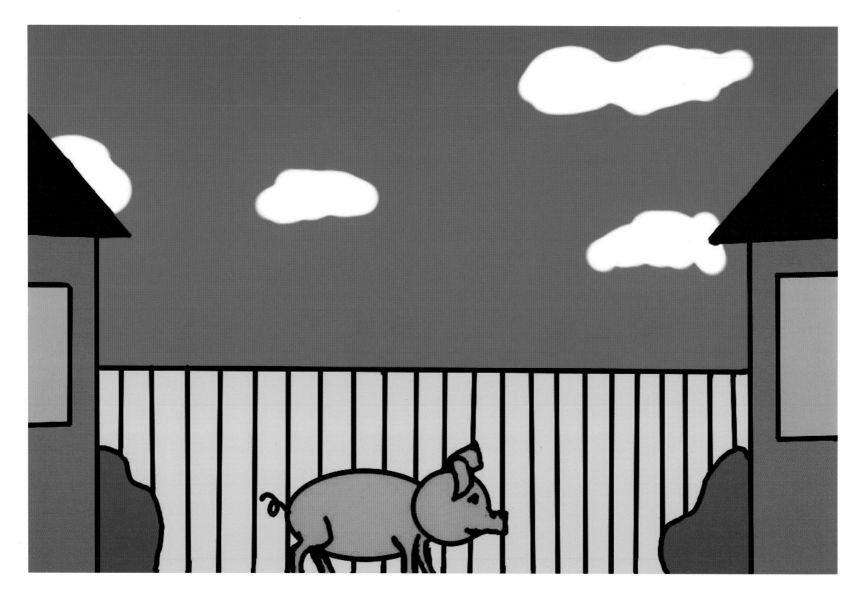

Arnold began to wander out of the yard in search of more food. He would visit the neighbors, singing his little oink song.

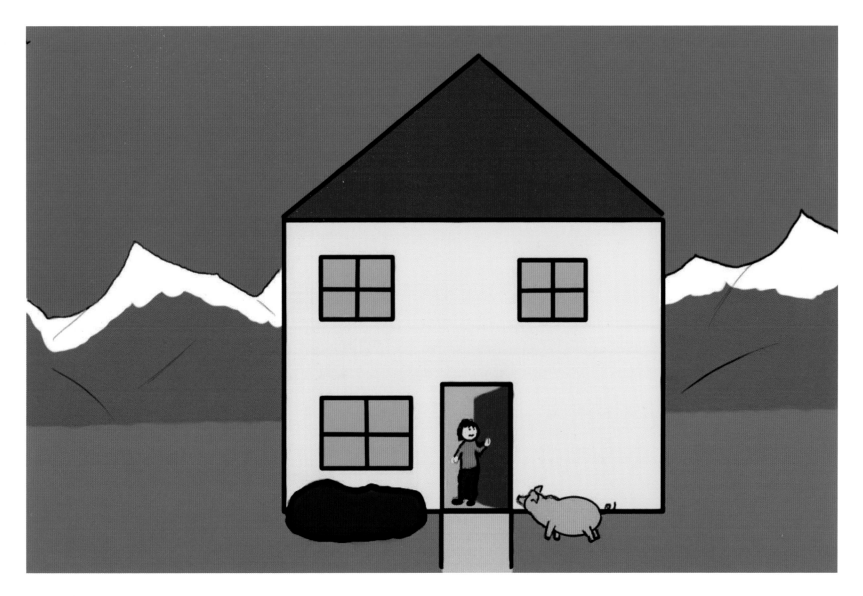

They thought he was such a cute little pig when he begged for food by oinking a little tune, so they gave him tacos, burgers, fries, and pizza. They laughed as he oinked with pleasure.

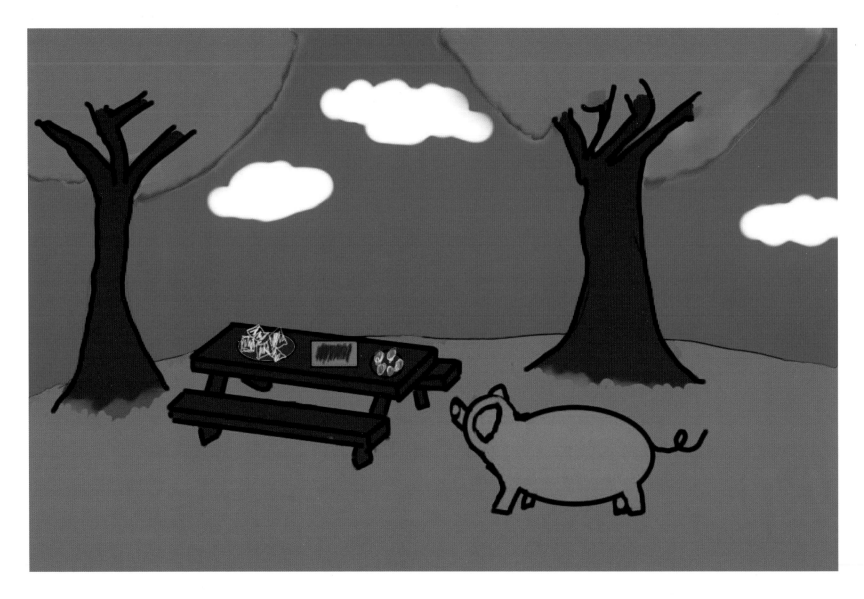

Arnold would go to the play ground and sing at picnics.
Mmmmm, he loved cake and ice cream. It made his mouth so
cold that when he oinked it came out as "yumyum oink".

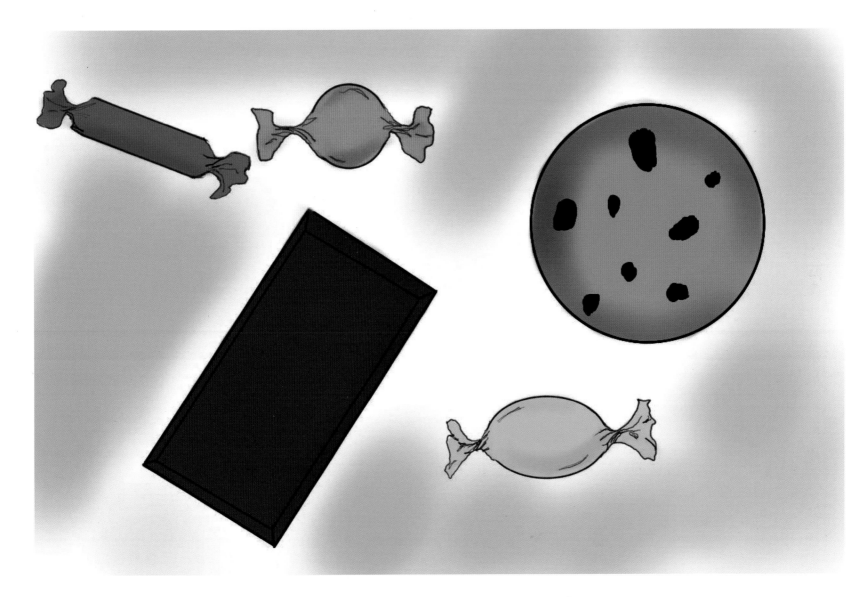

Arnold ate as much candy as he could find, especially chocolate.
He was so cute that people loved to give him cookies and candy to hear him oink with glee.

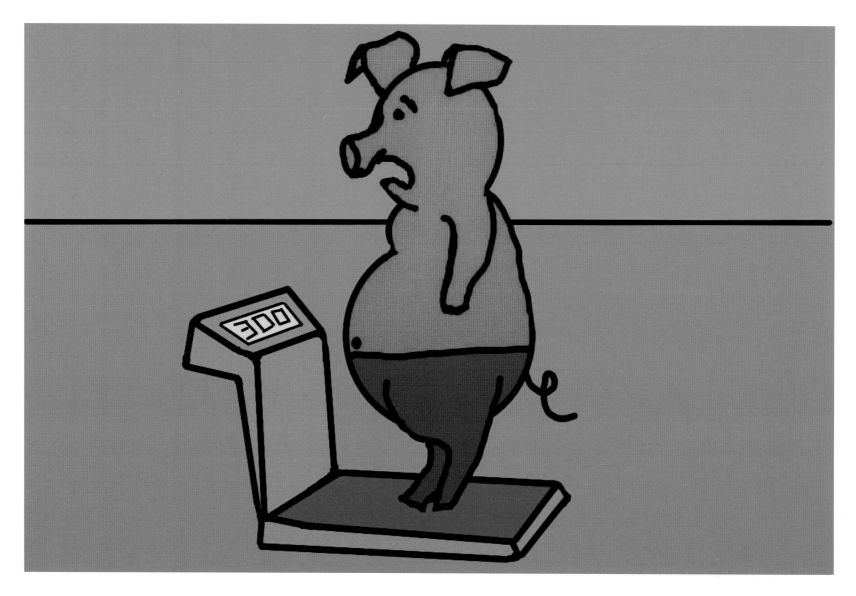

Arnold was such a cute little pig, but now he was getting to be a chubby little pig.

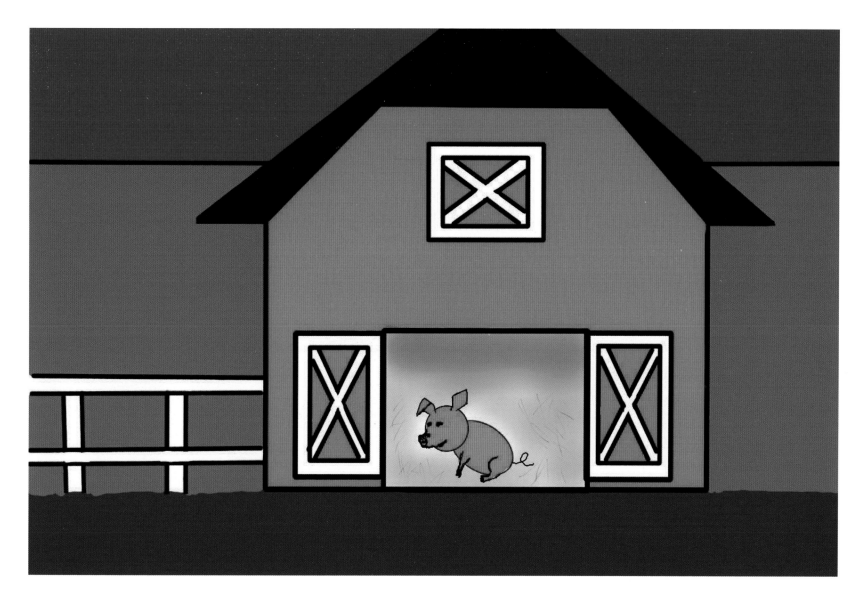

So Mom made him stay in the barn to keep him out of trouble.

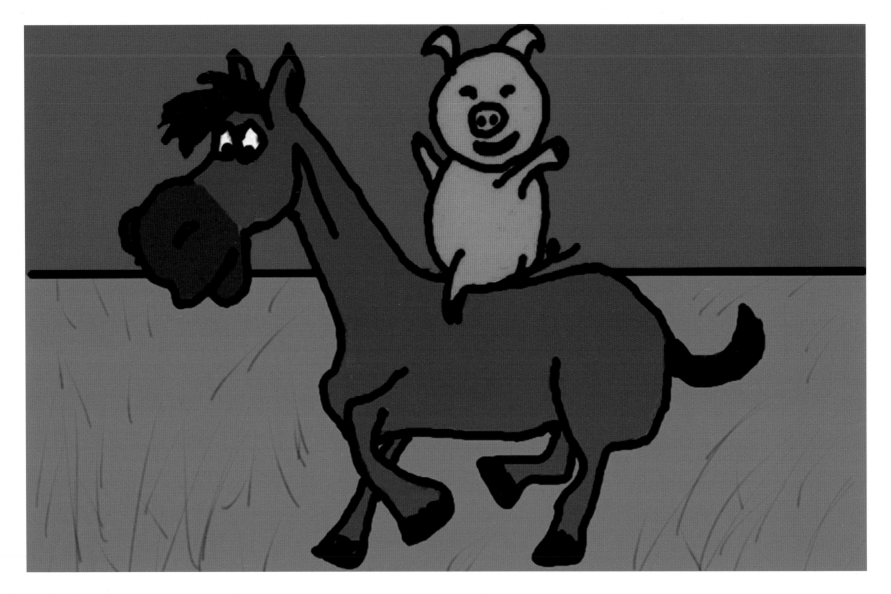

Arnold made friends with the horses. He was happy when they shared their oats, but oats were made for big horses, not little pigs.

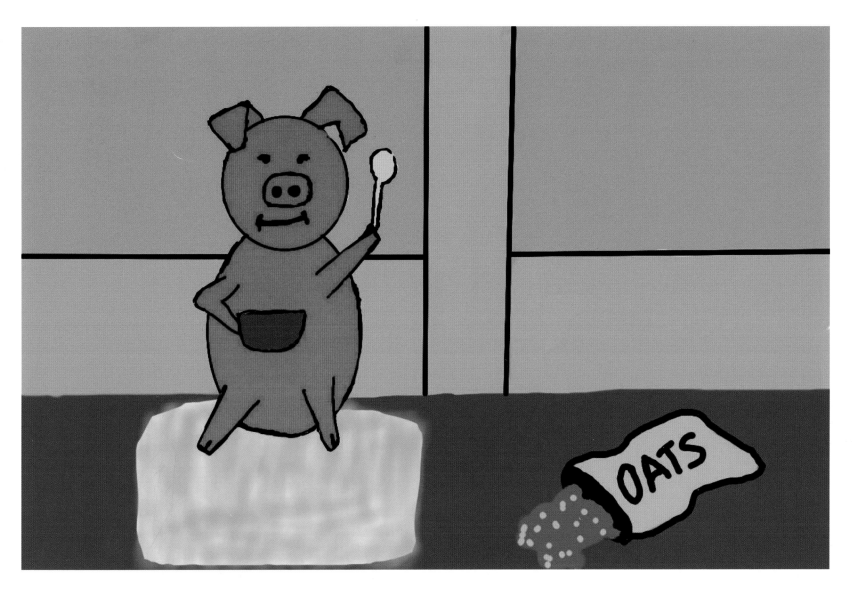

One night, Arnold was a naughty little pig and ate a whole bag of the horse's oats.

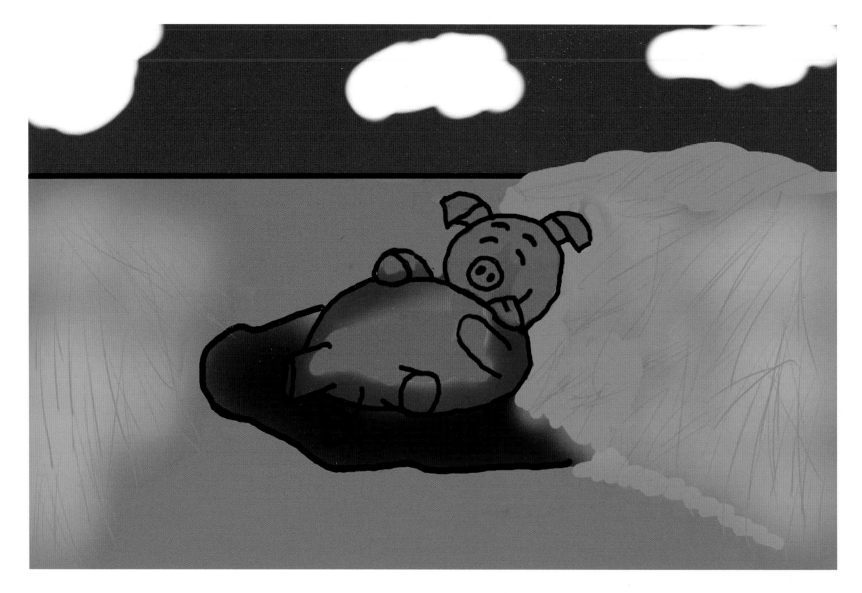

Arnold was so full he would not move. No matter how much we tried to get him up, he would not budge.

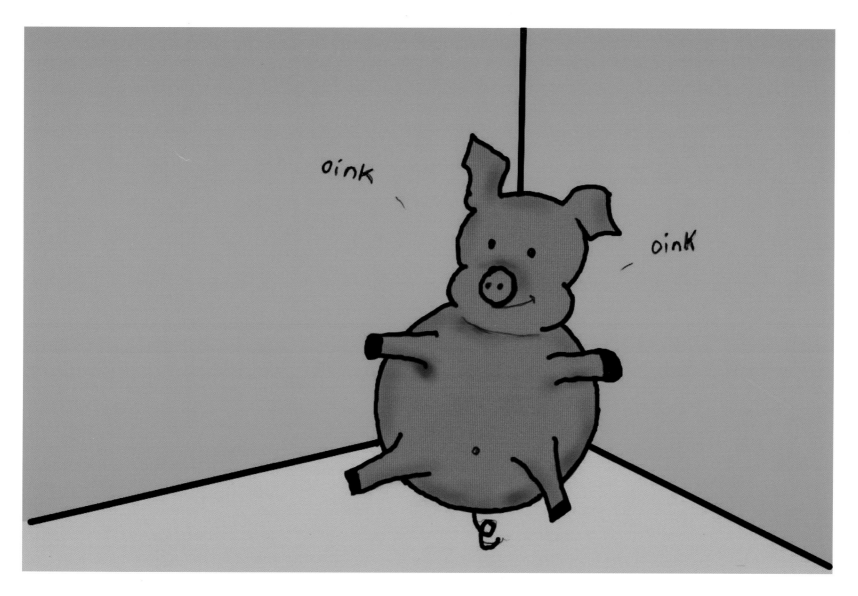

All he could do was lie there and let out a miserable little "Oink".
He could not sing a single oink song.

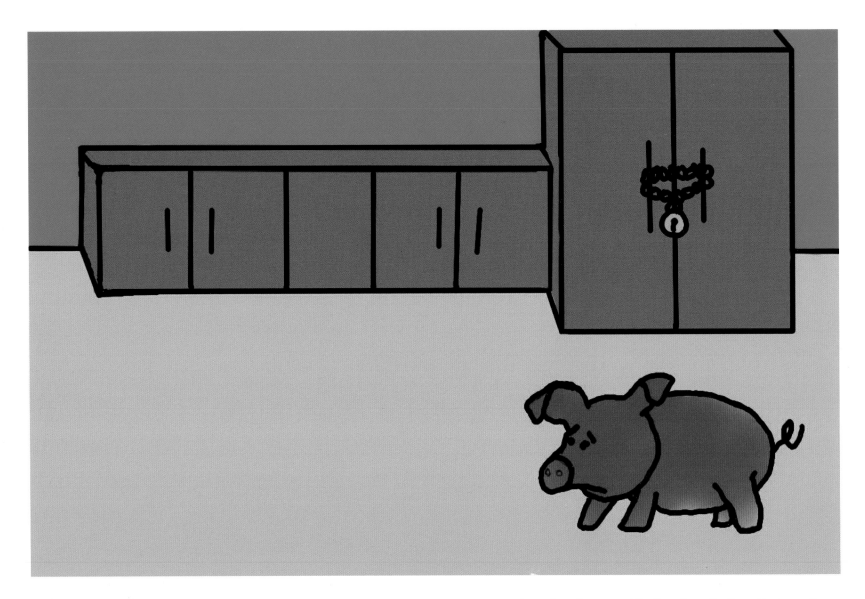

Arnold was such a mischievous little pig, that mom had to lock up all the junk food, trash, and oats because they were not good for cute little pigs to eat.

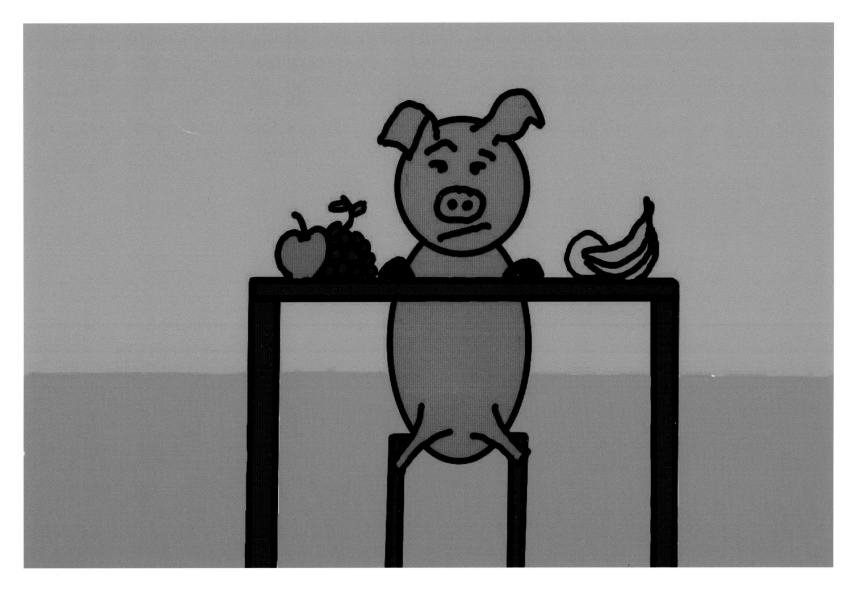

Instead, Mom gave Arnold fruits and veggies that were good for him to eat. Arnold was not happy. Mom said, "Try them, you'll like them".

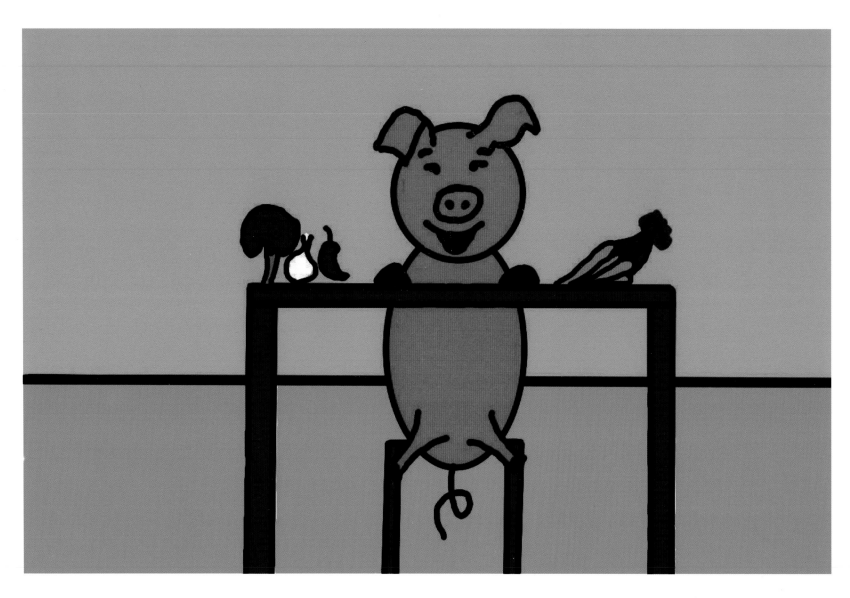

Arnold was very cute as he oinked and ate them. He did like them!
He wanted more fruits and veggies.
"Oink oink" he would sing to get more carrots.

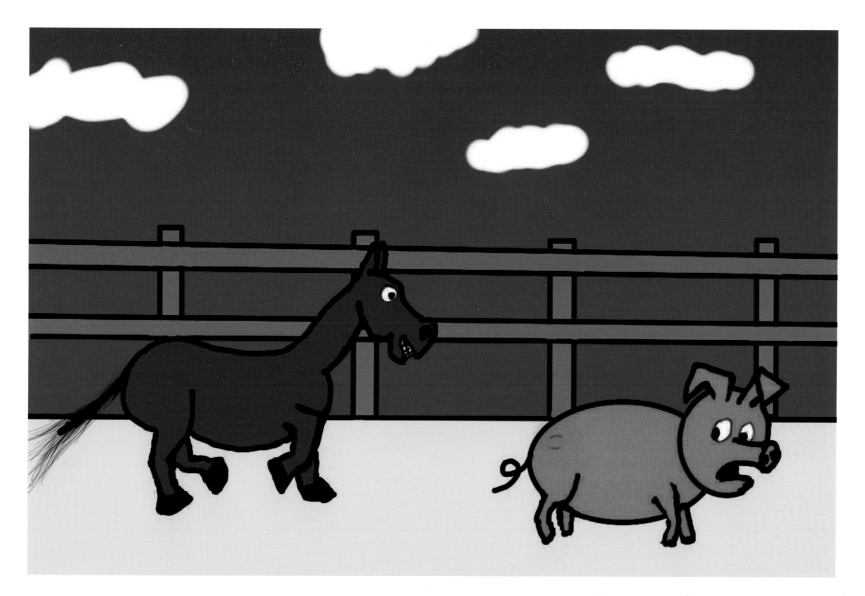

Mom also sent him to the corral to exercise with the horses.
The horses would chase him around the corral and bite his ham backside to make him run.
He did not like to run.

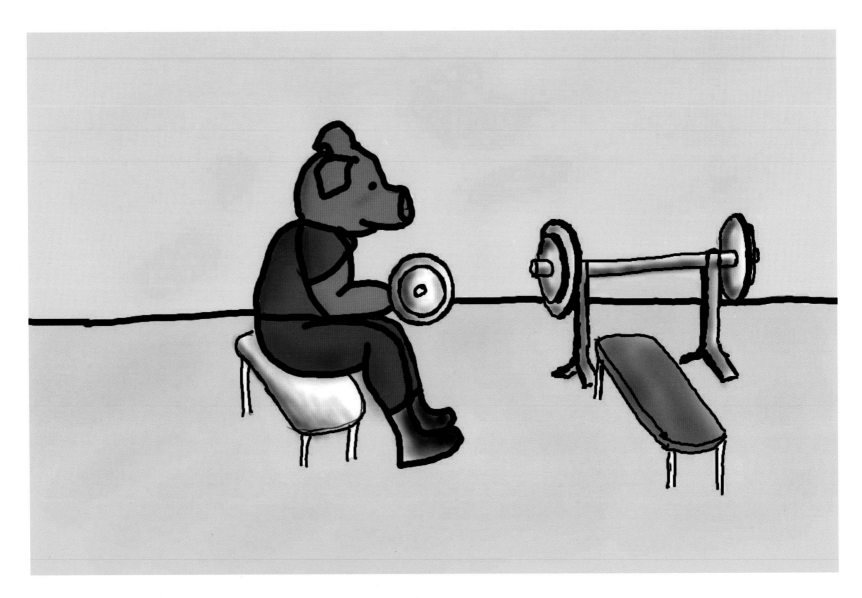

Arnold was now a cute healthy little pig.
He liked exercising!
It made him feel full of energy.

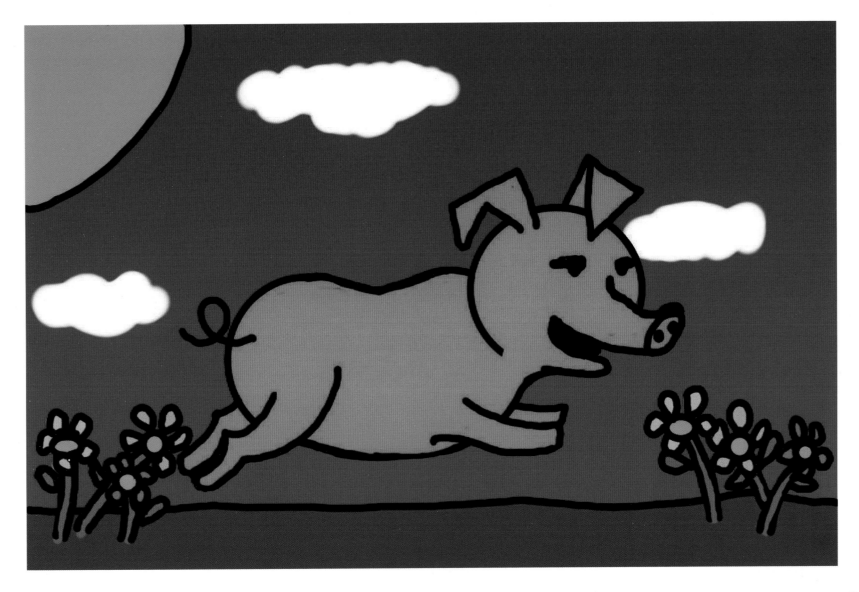

He could now run and play. He would sing his oink song with glee as he romped through the yard.
He liked running through the flowers to sing.
He liked to run in the grass and oink songs.

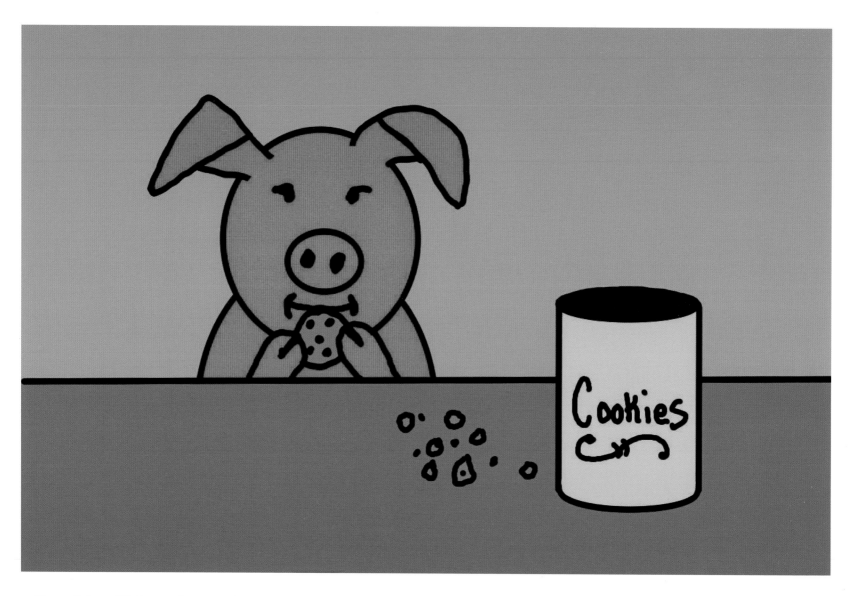

Arnold still loved cookies, but only once in a while, after dinner when he was not too full.

Who is the real Arnold?

Arnold was our cute little pet pig that really did like eating sweets and visiting the neighbors to oink for food.

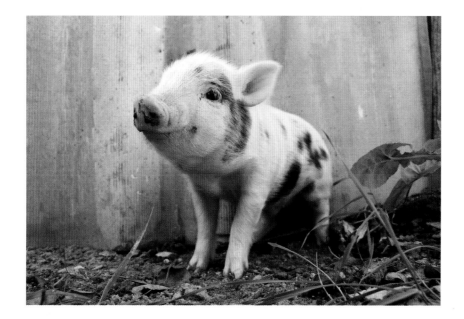

He would find his way into the corral where the horses would chase him and nip him in the rear.

However, as long as he stayed in the corral he would eat some of the horse's oats.

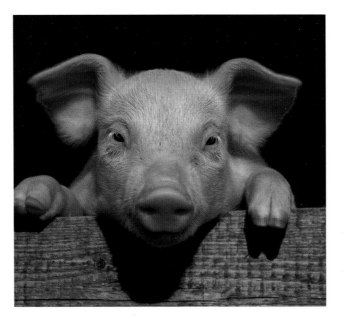

This is dedicated to Arnold our pet pig.
He learned that fruits and veggies are good for you.

Dog food is for dogs.
Horse food is for horses.

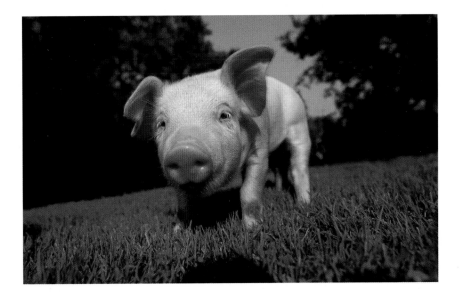

Cookies are a treat!

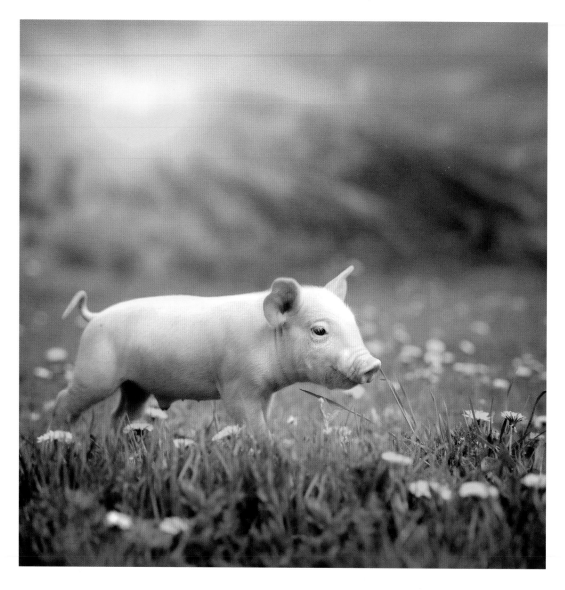

Arnold appeared on TV as part of his story. He delighted children as he sang his "oink" song.

Lisa Reinicke has appeared on local TV shows telling her original children's stories from her "Goodnights sleep collection" for children.

She lives in beautiful Colorado.

She has four grown children and five grandchildren who love to hear her read to them.

All of the stories originate to real instances in their lives.

"There is nothing more entertaining than real life lived to its fullest".

"A child in your arms and a book in your lap" is heaven.

Arnold was a good pig and loved his family very much.
He loved everyone and everyone loved him.
He would sing "oink" songs and play with the horses.
Arnold learned that veggies and exercise were good for him.